BE COMMANDO FIT

by James Latham

Table Of Contents

INTRODUCTION

I've seen it all before in this industry. How many fitness magazines have you read all suggesting a,b,c and promising x,y,z......how many of them have worked for you??

Imagine showing your ancestor from thousands of years ago a copy of last months Men's Health magazine telling him he needs to start bashing out oblique crunches to get the six pack he has always dreamed of...or he can't eat that fresh fish he has just caught because of the amount of fat it contains? The concept of "fitness" didn't even exist back then...it was the norm!

Health and Fitness is not a quick fix...it is not a fad...it is fundamental to human survival, which we seem to have neglected as time has passed. Thousands of years ago, if you were not fit.... you would die...fact. You would be incapable of hunting and incapable of avoiding hunters. Fast forward to today, where is the motive? I don't have to worry about saving my family from a saber tooth tiger...I barely have to get out of my f*****g pit to get my dry cleaning.

The things you will read in this e-book will clarify or perhaps contradict some of the things you may have seen or read in the past. For me the fitness industry has become full of tarts and testosterone loving meatheads whose definition of health and fitness is to arm curl their way to -5% body fat.

It never fails to amaze me the amount of people I see with chains, bands, belts, straps and corsets, yet cannot control their own bodyweight? People who swear by reverse keto intermittent carbohydrate back loading.... but are still shaped like pears?

.... If we don't enjoy it then it won't last. It is a lifestyle change. Therefore the aim of this e-book is to provide you with the essentials to staying fit and healthy by providing insight into how to workout efficiently, stay active and eat well....for life!

BE COMMANDO FIT

How on earth am I going to get fit enough to join the Royal Marines?????.....This is a question that I was faced with as a young boy. My decision to leave education and sack off the student life soon became reality when I decided to try and become a member of the fittest fighting force in the world. The aim of this e-book is to give you an insight into how I did it.... and what I learnt during my time as a Royal Marines Commando.

As a young 18 year old the only way, in my mind, to get fit was to pound the tarmac and cover as many miles as possible in a week and bash out as many press ups and pull ups as humanly possible....and yes it worked initially. Having ran mile after mile along the same stretch of road for 8 months without a clue about periodization, tapering or energy systems I found myself entering recruit training at a fairly substantial level.

One by one as the Royal Marines slowly chipped away at the recruits the weak began to separate and I found myself slowly sinking towards the bottom, but still in the pack. The way in which the Royal Marines define "fitness" is like no other. Realistically no other form of training will ever replicate recruit training apart from recruit training itself. No sick bastard is going to drag himself out of bed in the pissing rain at 0200 and go crawling through Woodbury common. Having said that, it taught me a lot...

As a now graduate in Sports, Health and Exercise Science, Level 3 personal trainer and currently studying towards a Masters degree in Strength and Conditioning, I realised my training could have been far more effective and so much more enjoyable.

Fitness is the ability to perform a certain task. For the Royal Marines that was the ability to carry your injured oppo (plus yours and his kit) into safe ground. The ability to march 30 miles across Dartmoor. The ability to control and manoeuvre your own body weight up ropes, over walls, through tunnels. It sounds hideous, however for me this should be standard across the entire population.

Granted, not everyone has access to the equipment that the military have in their armoury, but it isn't needed. The worst thrashings* of my life have all been on exercise with a just a hill to play with.

Today I can reflect on my experiences in university and couple it together with my time in the military to form a bulletproof, fool proof method to stay fit, healthy and robust, physically and mentally.

*thrashing – A term the Royal Marines use to describe getting worked physically until exhaustion

MINDSET

WHY?

When asked the key to getting fit and staying healthy, there is always one answer.... **Mind-set**. To which I usually receive a look of disappointment like they were after some sort of hidden secret that only people in the fitness industry know about. If there is a secret.... this is it!

Ask any Royal Marines Commando, past or present, what they found hardest going through training; the physical or mental aspect. I guarantee most of them will say mental. The same question kept repeating over and over in my head...why on earth am I putting myself through this?

You need to determine what is your "why". WHY are getting up at 0600 to pull heavy things off the floor? WHY are you spending at least one hour of valuable family time on machines that make me tired and nauseous? WHY have we decided to embark on this journey?

For me and every other Royal Marine it was the chance to earn the coveted Green Beret and become a member of the biggest, baddest boys club in the world. It wasn't the beret itself....i had about five of them during the time I was in corps...it was what it represented....it was my WHY!

Your "why" could be the ability to play with your children without having a defibrillator on standby. It could be feeling physically confident enough to walk around topless on holiday or perhaps the fear that your partner no longer finds you physically attractive.

Establish your "why"...and the rest becomes easy!

HOW?

Often the difficulty is getting started. For me this comes down to **routine** and **habit**.

"WE FIRST MAKE OUR HABITS, AND THEN OUR HABITS MAKE US"

- **John Dryden**

They say it takes 21 days to create a habit and 90 days to make a lifestyle. Habit defines us as human beings no matter how small or big it is. Having breakfast is a habit, brushing your teeth is a habit; all your weird little rituals are formed through habit. The same applies to diet and training...

Training has become such a big part of my life. So much that if I miss a day of training, it feels like something is missing and I get hit with an overwhelming sense of guilt. I have broken my habit! I have broken that thing that defines me as a person!

GETTING STARTED

- **Begin** training 2/3 days per week. Do not overload yourself and go from 0 to 6 sessions per week because that's what the ripped guy on Instagram does. You will burn out and subsequently fall out of love with the process.

- **LOVE** THE PROCESS: Enjoy it! If you hate running then don't run. If you hate chicken then don't eat it. Do something you enjoy and would like to do again. This could be a sport or a specific exercise or even a style of training.

- **Prepare** for the following day. Know what you are going to train and know how you are going to eat. Stepping into the unknown can cause you to fly so far out of routine that you will find yourself super setting calves with treadmill sprints and ordering 7 cheese burgers to go.

- **Manage** your time. I hate it when people say "I don't have time" or "I'm too busy". You can make no better investment in life than investing in yourself! As little as half an hour of physical activity each day can massively improve health and well being. Half an hour! And that is minimum! Why you wouldn't want to reduce disease and prolong life expectancy is beyond me.

BUILDING A HABIT

- **Timings.** Never be late. If you were late in the Marines the whole world would come down on you. This is a tradition engrained in the military. It is about discipline. If you are late it shows you don't care. It was never your priority. You are lax in your routine...and you will probably do it again. Make yourself accountable and make being on time your **habit.**

- Look **presentable**! Ever get that feeling that when you buy a new pair of shoes you can run ten times faster. Turn up every day looking clean and presentable and I promise you will perform better than if you just rolled out of bed and threw on your dirty washing.

PUSH YOURSELF

- Your body is an incredible machine. It will adapt to everything you throw at it. This can be an incredible weapon if used properly or it can be a very cruel mistress if abused. If you don't train and eat properly, your body will adapt by becoming sluggish, slow and fat! If you train.... your body adapts...if you OVERLOAD.... your body adapts more. This means that you need to push yourself EVERY session to keep your body guessing. It will overcome these hurdles by becoming stronger, faster and leaner!

- In the military we don't train to music. We are forced to self-motivate. I am not suggesting that you change the way you train if this works for you, but listen to your body! Get used to feeling tired and exhausted, it is totally normal. The "comfort zone" is a very difficult place to step out from but experiencing this in the gym has transferability into every day life. From hardships at work or even at home. Learn to control and embrace it!

DON'T BELIEVE THE HYPE

The media is an incredible learning tool, but sometimes this can be exploited. There is SO much information out there on health and wellbeing it is almost TOO much. I find people become so confused with the best way to do x,y,z that they literally throw all their books in the air and quit! When really it is so simple!

EVERYONE knows they need to be active. EVERYONE knows they need to eat well and EVERYONE knows what constitutes eating well. There are so many "diets" out there that choosing the right one sends peoples mind's into meltdown. If I were to recommend one book on diet it would be **"Food Rules" by Michael Pollan**. The book is probably the smallest and shortest I have ever read and not because he has NOTHING to say, but because there isn't much TO say. I will cover some of these rules later on in this e book along with other reliable sources of information.

TRAINING

For me, I like to think that humans can be stimulated through exploiting **8 key Fundamental Movement patterns:**

1. **Horizontal Push**
2. **Horizontal Pull**
3. **Vertical Push**
4. **Vertical Pull**
5. **Knee dominant**
6. **Hip dominant**
7. **Loaded carries**
8. **Core**

If you can walk out of a gym at the end of the week having smashed all of these movements then you have had a great week! I can think of nothing worse than walking into the gym knowing that all I have to look forward to training today is Deltoids or Calfs etc. The human body is an incredible machine, why not see how far it can go!

Now I am not suggesting that this is the ultimate body building protocol...because it isn't. If you want to look like Kai Green or Phil Heath then this book isn't for you. My style of training is efficient and "functional". You can still look very aesthetic through functional training whilst still maintaining a good quality of life and not wondering when your next tendon is going to snap!

EXERCISES

Here are some examples of the various types of human patterns. Each one can be exploited differently through training intensity. For example, I can get a cardio workout from the bench press if the weight was light enough and I could continually bang out repetitions for 5 minutes. Likewise I can turn it into a strength session if I used such a weight where I could only do 5 reps. It all depends on the load applied and the intensity you train at.

The examples below are some of the most effective exercises and movements we can use as humans to most effectively stimulate our bodies. Most of the exercises have derivatives that can act as a regression or progression based on skill level.

MOVEMENT	EXERCISE PROGRESSION		
	1	2	3
1. HORIZONTAL PUSH	HANDS ELEVATED PRESS UP*	PRESS UP	RING PRESS UP
	MACHINE CHEST PRESS	BENCH PRESS	
	FLOOR PRESS	DB CHEST PRESS	CHEST PRESS ON BALL
	SA FLOOR PRESS	SA DB CHEST PRESS	SA CHEST PRESS ON BALL
2. HORIZONTAL PULL	TRX ROW	INVERTED ROW	FEET ELEVATED ROW
	CABLE ROW	BENT OVER ROW (BOR)	PENDLAY ROW
	SINGLE ARM CABLE ROW (SEATED)	SINGLE ARM BOR	RENEGADE ROWS
	I,Y,T's	BANDED FACE PULLS	CABLE FACE PULLS
3. VERTICAL PUSH	SEATED PRESS	MILITARY PRESS	STANDING KB PRESS
	SEATED SHOULDER PRESS	SEATED SHOULDER PRESS (UNSUPPORTED)	SPLIT STANCE CURL-PRESS
	DB PUSH	PUSH PRESS	PUSH JERK

		PRESS	
		WALL BALLS (ADJUST WITH LOAD)	
4. VERTICAL PULL	BAND ASSISTED PULL UP	PULL UP	MUSCLE UP
	BANDED PULL DOWN	LAT PULL DOWN	SA PULL DOWN
	BANDED STRAIGHT ARM PULL DOWNS	STRAIGHT ARM PULL DOWN	BENT OVER CABLE ROW
	SEAT-STAND ROPE PULL		ROPE CLIMB
		MED BALL SLAMS (ADJUST WITH LOAD)	
	CLEAN PULL	HIGH PULL	DB SNATCH
5. KNEE DOMINANT	BOX SQUAT	BACK SQUAT	SKATER SQUAT
	GOBLET SQUAT	FRONT SQUAT	PISTOL SQUAT
	SPLIT SQUAT	LUNGE	WALKING LUNGE
	STEP UP	REAR LEG ELEVATED SPLIT SQUAT (RLESS)	BARBELL RLESS
	CLEAN PULL	POWER CLEAN	CLEAN AND JERK
	OVERHEAD SQUAT	POWER SNATCH	SNATCH

6. HIP DOMINANT	RACK PULL	DEADLIFT	DEFICIT DEADLIFT
	BACK EXTENSIONS	ROMANIAN DEADLIFT	SL RDL
		KB SWING (ADJUST WITH LOAD)	
	DOUBLE LEG GLUTE BRIDGE	SL GLUTE BRIDGE	GLUTE HAM RAISE
	GLUTE BRIDGE (ON HEELS)	HAMSTRING CURL	NORDICS
	BANDED GOOD MORNINGS	GOOD MORNINGS	SL GOOD MORNINGS

7. LOADED CARRIES		FARMERS WALK	
		SUITCASE CARRY	
		WAITERS WALK	
		OVER HEAD CARRY	
		FRONT RACK CARRY	
		ZERCHER WALK	
		BEAR HUG	

8. CORE	PLANK	SIDE PLANK	SIDE PLANK LEG ELEVATED
	FLR HANDS ELEVATED	FRONT LEANING REST	FLR ON RINGS
	ROLL OUTS	HAND WALK OUTS	STANDING ROLL OUT
		L SIT (ADJUST WITH LEG EXTENSION)	
	V SITS	BICYCLE KICKS	HOLLOW ROCK
	KNEE RAISES	LEG RAISES	TOES TO BAR
	DEAD BUG	BEAR CRAWL	LEOPARD CRAWL

11

* When regressing a press up I will always recommend elevating the hand rather than dropping to your knees so that you can maintain tension in your glutes.

FREQUENCY

Here's how you would structure your week, based around training frequency:

FREQUENCY	MOVEMENT PATTERN (No.)
1/week	**Try and hit all 6 patterns in the session**
2/week	Day1: 1,2,3,4, Day2: 5,6,7,8
3/week	Day 1: 5,6,7 Day 2: 1,2,8 Day 3: 5,6, 7
4/week	Day 1:1,4 Day 2:5,7 Day 3:2,3 Day 4:6,8
5/week	Day 1: 1,4 Day 2: 5,7 Day 3: 30-60 LISS* Day 4: 2,3 Day 5: 6,8
6+	Day 1: 1,4 Day 2: 5,8 Day 3: 30-60 LISS* Day 4: 6,7 Day 5: 2,3 Day 6: 1+2 or 3+4, 5 or 6

*Light Intensity Steady State cardio – Low-level cardio. Should be able to hold a conversation throughout.

STRENGTH		SIZE		CIRCUIT	
REPS	SETS	REPS	SETS	REPS	SETS
1 – 5 RM*	3-5	6 - 12 RM	2-4	12 +	FOR TIME*

*RM = REP MAX. 5RM would be the maximum weight you can lift for 5 repetitions. Therefore the fifth rep should be a major struggle and a spotter should always be used.

The above table can be used to dictate how many sets and reps should be conducted to perform each exercise. I would recommend beginning each session with either a Power or strength based movement whilst energy levels are at their highest.

An example week of training is detailed at the end of this book.

REST AND RECOVERY

Exercise is bad for you! Yep...it's bad for you. When you exercise you are causing trauma to your body. It is only when you recover that your body adapts to the trauma caused through exercise in hope that next time it can perhaps react stronger and faster. That is where the real gains lie!!

Sleep is the ultimate form of recovery. Hormones released during sleep cycles help the body to recover better than any ice bath or compression garment. 8 hours per night is recommended. However if you are anything like me I find this extremely difficult to achieve.

Here are a number of ways to get the best night sleep of your life:

- Turn of all electrical items 45 minutes before bed.

- Perform a household task. Spend a few minutes just tidying up your surroundings. Washing dishes, sweeping the floor etc. It provides some mental clarity and helps reduce stress that could ultimately keep you up at night.

- Write down tomorrow's tasks. Writing your tasks is therapeutic and can provide some peace of mind before entering the land of nod.

- Read a book. Rather than scrolling through social media, pick up a book and start reading, before you know it you'll be heads to z's.

- Reduce caffeine intake. I always consume my caffeine before mid day. That way there is absolutely no way it will keep me up later in the evening.

- High carb meals. Eating a meal rich in carbohydrates before bedtime will help you to sleep and no...it won't make you fat!

- Have a hot bath or hot drink (caffeine free of course). Increasing your core body temperature will help you to relax.

There are also other methods of recovery that you can use to help your body adapt and overcome a rough gym session.

- Proper diet and nutrition. Ensuring your body has all the right nutrients it needs is essential to recovery. The phrase "you are what you eat" is banded around everywhere and has almost been devalued, but it is so true. Don't starve your body of nutrients by feeding it junk food when it's crying out good, wholesome foods.

- Active recovery. Rather than sitting on the sofa and feeling sorry for yourself. Get up and get moving on your rest days. Let the blood flow around those sore limbs to get the blood and nutrients delivered to those places that need them the most. Take a walk or perhaps a swim, something low impact for 20-30 minutes.

TRAVEL GUIDE

Travelling is one of the biggest excuses to not keeping up with a health and fitness routine. Believe me some of the best workouts I have had have been on holiday. The sea and sand are some of the best places to workout...utilise it!

Travel Tips:

- Use body weight exercises. Body weight exercises are highly effective. Pick 5 of the following exercises...complete for 30 seconds, take 30 seconds rest between each exercise...and repeat 5 times...20 minutes... done!

- Press ups	- Mountain climbers	- Plank to press up
- Lunges	- Burpees	- Russian twists
- Plank	- Jump lunges	- V sits
- Squats	- Jump squats	- Squat thrust
- Down Up's	- Sit down stand up's	- Side plank

- Alcohol. Now I'm not saying go on holiday and not booze. Just be mindful, If you are going to drink, stick to lower calorie options such as Vodka + Tonic or Gin + Slim line. Just remember moderation is key and alcohol can be extremely bad for fat loss and recovery.

- Resistance Bands or Suspension Cables are great travel tools and pack really small. So if you want to really increase your training on holiday then make sure you pack one of these.

- Lacrosse/Hockey Ball. These little bad boys cause so much pain but are brilliant for self-message. After a long flight use a small but solid ball to really target those tight areas and release some of that built up tension.

NUTRITION

Diet seems to be the most misunderstood field in Health and Fitness. The amount of fad diets that appear left right and Chelsea leave people so confused they do not know which takeaway company to ring next. It is in fact VERY SIMPLE!

Forget macros and calories. How did my ancestors stay so lean without using macro-tracking apps? BECAUSE THEY ATE RIGHT! Tracking macros and calories seems to be the "In" thing right now. Unless you are trying to become the next Mr Olympia then don't bother. Everyone knows what he or she should be eating and everyone knows what he or she shouldn't be eating. Except everyone has now become so emotionally attached to food. Food has become a way of overcoming stress or tackling negativity, but ends up making it worse.

In "Food Rules" Michael Pollan fills his small book with the greatest, most honest comments about food: Live by these rules and you won't go wrong...

1. **"If it comes from a plant, eat it. If it is made in a plant, don't"** – Food that is made in a factory is bad for you. It's so basic yet people insist on eating ready-made meals that not even bacteria eats! If a bacterium doesn't want to eat it, then why should you?

2. **"Eat Food, Not a lot, Mostly Plants"** – Stick to a predominantly plant based diet. Fill your plate with as many vegetables as possible. Fibre is vital for burning fat and staying lean.

3. **"Don't eat anything your great-great grandmother wouldn't recognise as food"** – I love this quote! If I showed up at my nans house with a box of super noodles and a bag of bugles it would be straight in the bin. Think back to the dinners and lunches you used to have at your grandparents house...

4. **"Don't get your fuel the same place as your car does"** – Petrol station food is junk, don't eat it. If you know you are travelling long distances then prepare your meals before you leave.

5. **"Eat all the junk food in the world, as long as you cook it yourself"** – If you do have cravings for junk food then cook it yourself, that way you know every ingredient that goes into it. Plus you might even save a bit of dosh!

Example meal plans are shown at the end of this book.

If I were to recommend one book on nutrition it would be the one described above. The link is below if you want to purchase it!

http://amzn.to/2uaTXgr

EXAMPLE TRAINING PLAN

TYPE	EXERCISE	SETS	REPS	REST (seconds/mins)	WEIGHT (kg)	TEACHING POINTS
STRENGTH	BENCH PRESS	5	3 - 5	2 MINUTES	5RM	
HYPERTROPHY	A1. DB PRESS	4	8 - 10			SO THE NEXT FOUR EXERCISES ARE SUPERSETS. LABELLED A1 AND A2, B1 AND B2. THAT MEANS YOU DO ONE STRAIGHT TO THE NEXT WITH NO REST
	A2. BENT OVER ROW	4	8 - 10	90 SECONDS		FOR EXAMPLE YOU DO A1 THEN A2. REST AND REPEAT. ONCE YOU HAVE DONE 4 SETS MOVE ONTO B1 AND B2.
	B1.INCLINE CHEST PRESS	4	8 - 10			
	B2. SA DB ROW	4	8 EACH ARM	90 SECONDS		
	C1. FRONT LEANING REST	3	1 MIN	1 MIN		
FINISHER	250m ROW	6				1:1 WORK:REST

TYPE	EXERCISE	SETS	REPS	REST (seconds/mins)	WEIGHT (kg)	TEACHING POINTS
STRENGTH	SQUATS	5	5	2 MINUTES	5RM	DO 2 WARM UP SETS
	TRAP BAR DEADLIFT	4	6 - 8	2 MINUTES	8RM	
HYPERTROPHY	A1. WEIGHTED SPLIT SQUAT	4	8 EACH LEG		10KG EACH HAND	
	B1. GOBLET SQUAT	4	10			
	B2. RUSSIAN STEP UPS	3	12 / LEG	90 SECONDS		ADD DB IN EACH HAND IF NECESSARY
FINISHER	20 JUMP SQUATS				BODYWEIGHT	
	16 WALKING LUNGES				BODYWEIGHT	
	16 DB SNATCH	3 ROUNDS!			15KG	

TYPE	EXERCISE	SETS	REPS	REST (seconds/mins)	WEIGHT (kg)	TEACHING POINTS
STRENGTH	DEADLIFT	5	5	3 MINUTES	5RM	DO 2 WARM UP SETS
HYPERTROPHY	A1. RDL	4	8	2 MINUTES		
	B1. GLUTE HAM RAISE	4	10			
	B2. LUNGES	4	8 / LEG			ADD DB IN EACH HAND IF NECESSARY
	B3. KB SWING	4	30 SECS	90 SECS		
FINISHER	50M FARMERS WALK					
	10 BURPESS					
	20 THRUSTERS		9 MINUTE AMRAP			

*AMRAP - AS MANY ROUNDS AS POSSIBLE

TYPE	EXERCISE	SETS	REPS	REST (seconds/mins)	WEIGHT (kg)	TEACHING POINTS
STRENGTH	MILITARY PRESS	5	3 - 5	2 MINUTES	5RM	
HYPERTROPHY	A1. DB SHOULDER PRESS	4	8 - 10			
	A2. PULL UPS	4	8 - 10	90 SECONDS		USE ASSISTED IF NECESSARY
	B1. CURL - PRESS	4	8 - 10			
	B2. LAT PULL DOWN	4	8-10	90 SECONDS		
	C1. SIDE PLANK	2	30 SECS/SIDE	1 MIN		
FINISHER	DEADMILL SPRINTS	25 SECS	10	35 SECS		1:1 WORK:REST

EXAMPLE DIET PLANS

Below are just some typical examples of the standards of diet that would be expected to shred fat and become super lean. Obviously these are tailored to specific body weights however all can be adjusted accordingly through manipulation of proteins carbs and fats. As you can see meals are spread out across the day mainly to reduce hunger cravings and maintain blood sugar levels.

	SUNDAY	MONDAY	TUESDAY	WEDNESDAY	THURSDAY	FRIDAY	SATURDAY
MEAL 1	4 EGG OMELETTE WITH MIXED PEPPERS, 2 WITHOUT YOLK AND 2 WITH YOLK,	2 EGGS, SMOKED SALMON AND 1 SLICE OF WHOLEMEAL BREAD	OVERNIGHT OATS - 75G OATS, 50G GREEK YOGHURT, 200ML ALMOND MILK	4 EGG OMELETTE WITH MIXED PEPPERS, 2 WITHOUT YOLK AND 2 WITH YOLK,	4 EGG OMELETTE WITH MIXED PEPPERS, 2 WITHOUT YOLK AND 2 WITH YOLK,	4 EGG OMELETTE WITH MIXED PEPPERS, 2 WITHOUT YOLK AND 2 WITH YOLK,	4 EGG OMELETTE WITH MIXED PEPPERS, 2 WITHOUT YOLK AND 2 WITH YOLK,
MEAL 2	PROTEIN SHAKE, HANDFUL OF ALMONDS	PROTEIN SHAKE, HANDFUL OF ALMONDS	1 PIECE OF FRUIT AND A HANDFUL OF NUTS	PROTEIN SHAKE, HANDFUL OF ALMONDS	PROTEIN SHAKE, 1 PIECE OF FRUIT	1 PIECE OF FRUIT	LEAN MEAT, CLEAN CARB AND VEGETABLE BASED MEAL
MEAL 3	200G CHICKEN, 50G ASPARAGUS	150G STEAK, 75 GRAMS BROCOLLI AND CAULIFLOWER	200G CHICKEN, 125G BROWN RICE, 50G GREEN VEG	200G CHICKEN, 50G ASPARAGUS	SALMON FILLET, 150G SWEET POTATO, 50G GREEN VEG	150G WHITE FISH, 75G GREEN VEG	
MEAL 4	1 PIECE OF FRUIT AND HANDFUL OF NUTS	1 PIECE OF FRUIT AND 2 RICE CAKES	2 RICE CAKES, 1 TABLESPOON OF NUT BUTTER	1 PIECE OF FRUIT AND HANDFUL OF NUTS	1 PIECE OF FRUIT AND 2 RICE CAKES	HANDFUL OF NUTS	AT LEAST 1 PIECE OF FRUIT AND A SMALL HANDFUL OF NUTS THROUGHOUT THE DAY
WORKOUT							
MEAL 5	150G STEAK, 75 GRAMS BROCOLLI AND CAULIFLOWER	250G CHICKEN, 100G PASTA AND LIGHT HANDFUL OF CHEESE	150G STEAK, 200G WHITE POTATO, 50G VEG	150G STEAK, 75G VEGETABLES	CHICKEN/TURKEY SANDWICH ON WHOLEMEAL BREAD WITH A SALAD	ANY LEAN MEAT OR FISH WITH A GOOD PORTION OF VEGETABLES	CHEAT MEAL (ANYTHING YOU WANT)
MEAL 6 (OPTIONAL)	20G DARK CHOCOLATE 80%+ ONLY	20G DARK CHOCOLATE 80%+ ONLY	20G DARK CHOCOLATE 80%+ ONLY	20G DARK CHOCOLATE 80%+ ONLY	20G DARK CHOCOLATE 80%+ ONLY	20G DARK CHOCOLATE 80%+ ONLY	

*This meal is based on a 77kg Male with over 20% body fat

	MONDAY	TUESDAY	WEDNESDAY	THURSDAY	FRIDAY	SATURDAY	SUNDAY
MEAL 1	3 WHOLE EGGS, SPINACH, GRAPEFRUIT	4 EGG OMELETTE WITH MIXED PEPPERS, 2 WITHOUT YOLK AND 2 WITH YOLK,	3 WHOLE EGGS, SPINACH, GRAPEFRUIT	4 EGG OMELETTE WITH MIXED PEPPERS, 2 WITHOUT YOLK AND 2 WITH YOLK,	3 WHOLE EGGS, SPINACH, GRAPEFRUIT	3 WHOLE EGGS AND SPINACH	4 EGG OMELETTE WITH MIXED PEPPERS, 2 WITHOUT YOLK AND 2 WITH YOLK,
SNACK	100G CHICKEN, 50G AVOCADO, 50G GREEN BEANS	PROTEIN SHAKE, HANDFUL OF ALMONDS	100G CHICKEN, 50G AVOCADO, 50G GREEN BEANS	PROTEIN SHAKE, HANDFUL OF ALMONDS	100G CHICKEN, 50G AVOCADO, 50G GREEN BEANS	1 PIECE OF FRUIT	LEAN MEAT, CLEAN CARB AND VEGETABLE BASED MEAL
MEAL 3	100G TUNA 50 BROCCOLI	100G CHICKEN, 50G ASPARAGUS	100G TUNA 50 BROCCOLI	100G CHICKEN, 50G ASPARAGUS	100G TUNA 50 BROCCOLI	150G WHITE FISH, 75G GREEN VEG	
WORKOUT							
MEAL 4	100G STEAK 75G SWEET POTATO 50G GREEN VEG	150G STEAK, 75 GRAMS BROCOLLI AND CAULIFLOWER	100G STEAK 75G SWEET POTATO 50G GREEN VEG	150G STEAK, 75G VEGETABLES	100G STEAK 75G SWEET POTATO 50G GREEN VEG	ANY LEAN MEAT OR FISH WITH A GOOD PORTION OF VEGETABLES	CHEAT MEAL (ANYTHING YOU WANT)

*DAYS IN BOLD ARE TRAINING DAYS
* ALL WEIGHTS ARE MEASURED WHEN COOKED

*This meal plan is based on a female weighing between 55-65kg with +25% body fat.

SMART CHOICES

CLEAN CARBS	PROTEIN	FATS
Brown Rice	Chicken	Coconut Oil/ Olive oil
White Rice (Post workout)	Steak	Avocado
Sweet potato	White Fish	Almonds
Quinoa	Lentils	Dark Chocolate (<20g)
Oats	Turkey	Eggs
Brown Bread	Salmon	Grass fed butter

SNACKS
FRUIT X 1 portion
NUTS X Handful
PROTEIN SHAKE
PROTEIN BAR X 1
GREEK YOGHURT
DARK CHOCOLATE (20g)
BOILED EGG X 2

Supplements

A lot of supplements can be extremely expensive so I do not like prescribing an extensive list of dietary supplementation. If a healthy and balanced diet is maintained then supplements should be limited.

Whey Protein: Find a protein powder that has a good reputation as well as a good level of macronutrient breakdown. This should be consumed immediately after your morning workout and then perhaps once throughout the day between meals. This will essentially help rebuild your muscles after extensive periods of stress.

Multi Vitamin – Any multi-vitamin from a pharmaceutical company will be fine. Consume this in the morning only. This will ensure that despite your balanced diet you have a steady source of your body's essential vitamins.

Fish Oils (Omega 3) – This will predominantly aid in joint health and repair. Omega 3 has also been shown to increase the efficiency of the body's nervous system whilst lowering blood pressure and cholesterol.

BOOKS AND REFERENCES

The list below is a list of books that I would highly recommend if you are looking to broaden your knowledge in exercise and health. I have hand picked them myself having read them all. I hope you get the same pleasure reading them as I did.

AUTHOR	TITLE	PURPOSE
MICHAEL POLLAN	FOOD RULES	DIET AND NUTRITION ADVICE
JULIAN GOATER	THE ART OF RUNNING FASTER	IMPROVE RUNNING CAPACITY
PAUL CHEK	HOW TO EAT, MOVE AND BE HEALTHY	OVER ALL TRAINING AND DIET ADVICE
KELLY STARRETT	BECOMING A SUPPLE LEOPARD	MOBILITY AND JOINT HEALTH
JOE WICKS	LEAN IN 15	HEALTHY FOOD RECIPES

I HOPE YOU ENJOYED THIS BOOK...PLEASE LEAVE A REVIEW ON AMAZON IT IS GREATLY APPRECIATED

www.ingramcontent.com/pod-product-compliance
Lightning Source LLC
Chambersburg PA
CBHW061951280526
45787CB00004B/1813